Romantic Dreams

Romantic Dreams and Treatment

Contents and points :-

- Romantic dreams.
- Treatment without medicine.
- Romantic dream is a very sadness thing and shameful thing.
- It is a very simple disease so don't worry.
- It is curable within some days.
- How to take care while sleeping.
- Brain, heart and mind.
- Daily duty and work.
- Love affairs.
- Enemies.
- House and village.
- Money problem.

Romantic Dreams

Generally most of the people are facing this romantic dream disease problem. This disease is not a dangerous disease but it is a very shameful disease of all people. If people are sleeping in deep sleep at night, then they are looking dreams. But what is this romantic dream. Any people can see this romantic dreams. If people are doing any love affairs with others then they can see romantic dreams while sleeping. But it is a wrong statement. If you are not doing any love affairs, then you can also see romantic dreams while sleeping. A completely healthy people can also see romantic dreams while sleeping. If you are looking romantic dreams while sleeping, at that time if you feel sex feeling, then a liquid will out from your sex part, so it is the problem. You are not doing sex, but you are feeling sex while looking romantic dreams. There are many causes that you can see romantic dreams. The romantic dream is not the problem. There is another problem in your body, so you are looking romantic dreams. It is not a bad thing to see romantic dreams, but it is the problem if the liquid outs from sex part while looking romantic dreams while sleeping. It is possible to solve completely this romantic dream disease problem. It is possible to become curable completely from this romantic dream disease. Don't worry if you are looking romantic dreams while sleeping, but we will do such things as the liquid will not out from sex part while looking romantic dreams while sleeping. Too much of everything is bad. So if you see too much dreams while sleeping then it is bad. If you are going latrine once or twice in a day then it is not a disease, but if you are going latrine ten times in a day then it is a disease. Then you have to contact with a doctor immediately to take medicine to stop this disease to go latrine many times in a day, if not you can die. It is a very simple example. Exactly if you are looking too much dreams while sleeping, then you have to contact with a doctor immediately. But sometimes you are looking dreams within some days gap, then no problem. Again if you are looking romantic dreams sometimes then it is also not a problem, but if the liquid outs from sex part while looking romantic dreams then it is the problem. We will solve this problem as the liquid will not out form sex part while sleeping even while looking romantic dreams. Then problem is solved. You can see romantic dreams but the liquid will not out, then problem is finished. I can say that a doctor can not solve this simple problem romantic dream of you. Again this simple problem can not be solved by taking medicine. If you will take medicine for this simple problem, then there can be side affect of medicine in your body. So this romantic dream problem can not be solved by medicine. Some people are getting up early in the morning to solve this romantic dream problem. They get up at 4am early in the morning. But it is not the exact solution of this romantic dream problem. You can get up at 10am, it is not a problem. If you have no work tomorrow, then you can sleep up to 10am. It is not a problem. There is not required to get up early in the morning. You can get up at 6am or 7am or 8am at any time up to you feel comfortable. But it is also a good habit to get up early in the morning before sun rise and it is also good for health. But to get up early in the morning is not the exact solution to solve the romantic dream disease problem. Because you can see romantic dreams at any time after sleeping. You can see romantic dreams, just after sleeping or after 1 hour or after 2 hour or at the time sun rise or just before get up. Again you can see this romantic dreams if you are sleeping in day time. If some people are doing night duty and they are sleeping in day time. Then think what is the get up timing those who are sleeping in day time if required. So sleeping timing is not affect to your romantic dream problem. Then you can sleep at any time and you can get up at any time, it is not a problem. Main problem is that if you are looking romantic dreams while sleeping means there is a **wound or infection inside your brain surely,** because of any cause by our outside activities. There is a problem in your brain, so you are looking romantic dreams. But it is your work to keep safe to your brain, to give protection to your brain, to take care properly of your brain. Because your brain have some problems, so you are looking romantic dreams. But why the brain have problem. It can not possible that because of which reason the brain wound or brain infection had started. But it is possible to become curable completely from this brain wound or brain infection disease. You can remember to your past life, that because of which cause the brain wound or brain infection had started and for which you are looking the romantic dreams while sleeping and liquid out. There are many uncountable problems that can affect to your brain. As heavy work pressure can affect to your brain. It can be heavy physical work pressure or heavy official work pressure. If you are fighting or quarrelling with others, then it will also affect to your brain. If they scold or rebuke you and if they beaten you, then it will also affect to your brain. If you will do unnecessary arguments with your enemies, then it will also affect to your brain. All these are affecting to your brain. Again you are going alone and a dog will bark near you loudly, then it will also affect to your brain. There are many causes that can affect to your brain. So take care of your brain properly always as anything will not affect to your brain at any moment. If your brain remains safe then you will never see romantic dreams. Again even if you will see romantic dreams then the liquid will not out from sex part, if your brain is safe. So it is our work to keep safe to our brain from outside affects, then the romantic dream disease problem will be solved.

But if you have this romantic dream disease then you have to take care for some days, while just going to sleeping, so try to sleep comfortably with good pillows and remember that if your brain is safe today from outside affects or not. Then within some days this disease is will be curable completely. Again if you have this romantic dreams disease then you have to keep distance to yourself from any romantic works. If you will do heavy work in day time again you will do romantic work, both are not possible at a time, if you will do both work then it will affect to your brain surely. Because human brain has **limited capacity**. If your brain is affected by this work then you will **surely** look romantic dreams while sleeping and liquid out **surely**. If you do any love affairs or any romantic works in day time, then don't do any other heavy work. Because work pressure and love affairs, both are **not possible**, then it will affect to the brain. Again if you are doing heavy physical work and if you are doing heavy mental work or official work. Both physical work and mental work are **not**

possible to do at a time, then it will affect to your brain. If it is your habit to do office work then do your office work. If it is your habit to do physical work then do your physical work. But if you will do both work then it will affect to your brain **surely**. So it is our work to keep it **attention** always as any type of outside works or problems will not affect to our brain. Then try to keep safe to your brain from outside affects. It is required to keep distance from bad people, to keep distance from noise, try to sleep in separate bed room etc.. Some people are there who try to **hurt** to your mind and heart always by talking method or fighting method, so if their activity will affect to your brain then it will become romantic dreams **surely** while sleeping and liquid out from sex part **surely**. It is good to keep distance from this type of people and don't fight with them. Because they **can know clearly** that how to hurt to the mind and heart of people which will cause the romantic dream problem and liquid out. So it is their habit to hurt to other people. There are some other causes of this romantic dream problem and liquid out. If you are cutting hair once in a month then you can face a problem while cutting hair. That problem is that if the barber touching or robbing the comb with **your ear** many times, then it will affect directly to your brain. Because the top corner of the ear is also a soft and sensitive part of the body. All the barbers **can know** about this thing but they always try to rub or touch the comb many times to the ear corner while cutting hair of people. So keep it **attention** that as the barber will not touch the comb to your ear at all while cutting hair and say to the barber before start hair cutting as the comb will not touch **to the ear**. Only bad barbers are doing this type of activity. There are good barbers who can cut hair in very smooth. It is our work to keep **attention** as any type of incident or accident will not affect to our brain. If brain will be affected then it will be the cause of romantic dreams and liquid out **surely**. Because brain is the softest element of the body. We can not see brain out side of the head but there is a brain inside the head. As we can not see the heart but there is a heart inside our chest. As we can not see the kidney but there is a kidney inside our waist. So it is our work to keep **attention** as any type of work or any type of incident will not affect to our brain. If brain will remain safe then we will **enjoy** our life full. If brain will remain safe then you can **enjoy** your love life with others. But think that too much of everything is bad, so too much of love affairs is also bad, because it will also affect to brain, then again romantic dreams and liquid out **surely**. So you can move in love affairs but keep it **attention** as it will not affect to your brain. Because too much of everything is bad. Those who have this romantic dream disease, then their life will be muddy, as they will feel wallowing in mud. Those who are doing sex related real crime they can not affected by this type of romantic dream disease, but those who are good people, they are affected by this romantic dream disease, but why. Because they **can not** take care of their brain properly though they are good people. So it is our work to take care of our brain properly, to keep safe to our brain properly, as any type of activities will not affect to our brain.

If you are doing love, after get success in love, you can do sex, it is not a problem. But keep it attention that as this love and sex activities will not affect to your brain. If your brain is affected then you will see **surely** the romantic dreams and liquid out while sleeping

surely. So keep it **attention** always that, as any type of your activity or others activity will not affect to your brain. You can use condom while doing sex, because sexual disease will not transfer, again you will not be pregnant if liquid out. It is a bad thing to do abortion after become pregnant. So keep it attention that as liquid will not out while doing sex. Again if your brain will be **affected** while doing sex then you will see romantic dreams while sleeping and liquid will out **surely**. So it will be **our aim** as liquid will not out while doing sex and in **romantic dreams** while sleeping. So keep it **attention** properly to take care of brain. Then we can **enjoy** our life really.

Sometimes you can feel that your heart is weak. It is also a reason of romantic dreams and liquid out, if your heart is weak. But if you feel the weakness in heart, then get up early in the morning and go to morning walk and slow running, do light exercise etc.. If you have more work pressure then take a leave from work and stay inside house and take rest. If required go to move in distance new places in visit. Then your heart and mind **will remain fresh**. Again eat good foods and try to sleep comfortably with good pillows. Then heart weakness problem can be solved easily, but you have to take care of your brain as anything will not affect to your brain, so keep it **attention** about brain safety. Then within some days the romantic dreams with liquid out problem will be solved. If your brain remain safe then you will never face this romantic dream and liquid out problem while sleeping. So it is **your work** it is **your duty** always, to take care of your brain properly as anything activity will not **affect** to your brain.

If your romantic dream and liquid out problem is solved, then **what will you do**. If you will move in love affairs, then it is not a problem. But think that the human life is not a permanent life. Death, old age, disease etc. will come in our life surely. You will die surely, I will die surely and we all will die one day surely. So try to keep distance from sex related things and romantic works and try to live in **peaceful life**. Then you will reach near to the permanent life where there is no death, no old age, no disease etc.. Then this permanent life will be most enjoyable. Think that **where** is this permanent life, that is no death, no disease, no old age.

What is this dream that you can see while sleeping. Again who controls to this dream. It is a very difficult task to know details about this dream. Again romantic dreams. If you want to do research about this dream, then write down the dream in your diary everyday, that you can remember the dream after get up. Then one day will come, you will get many secret information about dreams. There is no need to talk about this dreams with others, only try to write down.

If you are looking romantic dreams while sleeping in some days interval and liquid out, then **don't worry**, it is possible to become curable from this disease **completely**. If you will not take care of your body properly, then this disease will become more **critical**. Again if you are looking romantic dreams daily and liquid out daily then it is a very **dangerous situation**. Then you have to spend more money to go in visit to distance new places to become curable form this disease **immediately**. If your brain is affected because of any dangerous conflict or fighting with your enemies, then you can see many romantic dreams while sleeping and liquid out **many times** while sleeping. This is the **most** critical situation. So take care of your brain properly as any outside incidents will not affect to your brain. If not you have to contact with a doctor immediately. But it is our work to take care of our body properly and to take care of our brain properly. **Very simple** as we take care of our eye, as we take care of our ear, as we take bath daily, as we go latrine daily, as we do brush to clean teeth, **exactly** we will take care of our brain always. There are some bad people who always try to hurt to your brain, but it is our work to **keep distance** from this type of people. This type of bad people can do **anything,** even they can do rape or murder of you. Because they are doing secret preplanning to attack you before many days, but you can not aware about this. They have the knowledge that how to create romantic dream disease problem by hurting to your brain or heart or mind. But you have **no knowledge** about this romantic dreams, so you are affected by this type of bad people. It is good to keep distance from this type of bad people. Again heavy work pressure can be the cause of this romantic dreams, because heavy work **affects** to our brain. If a dog is barking near you loudly, then will **affect** to your brain. If you are moving in love affairs **too much**, then is will also **affect** to your brain. So it is our work to keep **attention** always as anything outside activity will not affect to our brain. It is our work to **keep safe** to our brain. Then romantic dream and liquid out problem will be solved **completely** within some days.

What is brain? There is a brain inside our head, that is a muscles. This brain is a softest element of the body. So it is our work to **keep safe** to our brain, it is our work to **take care** of our brain properly. Sometimes while playing we injured with our foot and we can walk at all. We think that bone of the foot is broken. If the bone is not broken after contact with a doctor or after doing x-ray, but we feel **very pain** and we can not walk at all. Then what is this problem if you can not walk. Because the injury is in the muscles in our foot. So you can not walk. **Exactly** there can be injury inside brain, because brain is also a muscles. If there is an injury in foot muscle, then we can not walk up to 15 days or more days. In this situation if you try to run, then think what will happen the **condition** of your foot. So you have to take rest for some days **completely** up to the foot injury will become curable. **Exactly** if the brain muscle have injured then you have to **take rest** also for some days. If you are looking romantic dreams and liquid out while sleeping, then think that **it is brain injury or infection**. So you have to take care properly of your brain **for some days** to become curable **completely**. If you can not take care of your brain properly then this brain injury or infection will create **critical situation**. As in foot injury if you will try to run then you can become lame, then whole life will become sorrowful. So it is our work if you are looking romantic dreams and liquid out, then it is the reason of **brain wound or infection**, then it is our work to become curable from this brain wound or infection. There are different many causes of brain injury, as there are different many reason of foot injury. But it is our work to become curable from this brain injury and to take care of our brain properly to become curable, if the brain is affected. Then it is possible to solve the romantic dreams and liquid out problem while sleeping **completely** within some days.

Now a days film or cinema affects to our mind and brain. But really film or cinema has no affect to our mind and brain. Too much of everything is bad, so too much looking of cinema or film is also bad. Mainly romantic scenes of film or cinema is affecting to us, but really it is not affecting to us. If you think that it affects to us, then remove your eye from romantic scenes and don't look to this romantic scenes of cinema or film. Don't see the romantic videos in website, cinema or film. Sometimes romantic scenes are useful to some people as a medicine. So they are looking this romantic scenes. If there is no required then don't see these romantic videos or scenes in cinema or film or website. It is the question, that why are they creating romantic scenes in film or cinema. Some people can say that the film makers are creating romantic scenes to earn more money from people, as many people will be attractive to see films. It is the reason that the film makers are creating romantic scenes in films. But there are many other causes to enter, romantic scenes inside the film or cinema, so you can ask details about this to film hero heroine of films. But it is the **problem** as we will not see romantic dreams and no liquid out while sleeping. Then it will not be the **problem** if you see film or cinema. This film or cinema has started within last 100 years. Then think before hundred years, before thousand years, people have also this romantic dream and liquid out problem while sleeping. Before 100 years before 1000 years, there was no cinema or film, but people of this time were also **affected** by this romantic dream and liquid out problem while sleeping. So people of this past time were also trying to get up early in the morning at 4am before sun rise. It is not the **exact** solution of this romantic dream disease to get up early in the morning. If your brain is **safe** then you can get up at any time at 6am or 7am or 8am at any time up to you feel comfortable. But it is good for health to get up early in the morning before sun rise. But to get up early in the morning, it is not the solve of romantic dreams and liquid out problem while sleeping.

I want to solve your romantic dream and liquid out problem while sleeping. After you become curable form this romantic dream and liquid problem then you can do anything love affairs and sex relation, it depends upon your **personality**. If you will move in love affairs or sex relation then it is your personality, it is your desire, it is your future. But keep it **attention** that anything that you can do love or sex, as that will not **affect** to your brain. If your brain will be affected then you will see romantic dreams and liquid out **surely**. Now a days the condom is very useful while doing sex with your lover. It is the modern age, the science is going developed very fast. So it is not a problem to you to use condom while doing sex with your lover. The sex related disease will not be transfer and the sex part will remain safe if you will use condom while doing sex with your lover. Before many years ago we are using wooden cart to go one place to another place, but now a days we use aeroplane to go one place to another place. Because the science is developed. So use of condom is also not a bad thing while doing sex with your lover in this modern age of science. But keep it attention that as liquid will not out while doing sex and as brain will not be **affected** while doing sex. If brain will be affected while doing sex then romantic dream and liquid out **surely** while sleeping. So keep it **attention** that as anything activity will not **affect** to your brain, if brain is affected then romantic dream and liquid out **surely** while sleeping. So **take care** of your brain properly and try to **keep safe** to your brain. It is the **duty** and **responsibility** of everyone, to take care of brain. Because the human brain has **limited** capacity. So if the brain will do anything out of capacity, then the brain will be affected, the brain will be injured, then the wound or infection will start inside brain. Again brain is the smooth and softest element of the body. If any problem starts inside brain then romantic dream and liquid out **surely** while sleeping. So take care of brain always as a daily duty and routine.

If brain remain **alert** then anything can not affect to brain. But some people try to hurt to your brain if you are not alert. They can understand your **alertness** and they start to attack to your brain or mind. Because they are the thief, they are the criminal. They always think that your mind is alert or not, then they start attack to your brain, then a **wound or infection** will start inside your brain. A thief can think about the alertness of a people and as the thief can make preplanning before start stealing.

If you have any work pressure, then take **special care** while sleeping. Sit down in a **comfortable chair** for half an hour before go to bed. Then go to bed to sleep comfortably with good pillows. But if any work pressure affects to your brain, then the romantic dream and liquid out **surely** while sleeping tonight. **So it is your work to keep it attention as anything activity will not affect to your brain at all.** Reading and Writing is also a hard work, if you are **writing** something remembering anything deeply then it will also affect to your brain. If someone will say you **tension word** while go to sleeping, then it will also affect to your brain. So try to sleep **alone** in a separate bed room.

If you will do heavy work and you will try to get up quickly early in the morning before sunrise in the fear of romantic dream and liquid out, **it is not the rule.** Always try to take care of your brain as anything activity will not affect to your brain at all, **it is the rule.**

If someone will **disturb** you by talking while you are doing research or deep thinking then **it will also affect** to your brain surely. If brain will be affected then romantic dream and liquid out **surely** while sleeping. So it is good to keep **distance** from bad people as they will not disturb in your work.

Don't do sex with your lover, it is good. Because if brain will be affected while doing sex, then romantic dream and liquid out **surely** while sleeping. Again if you will do sex with your lover then keep it **attention** as liquid will not out and as brain will not be affected. I want to say that if you are thinking and trying to do sex, then it is a **deep research.** So while you are doing this love or sex **research,** if anyone will **disturb** you by talking or anything activity, then it will affect to your **brain** surely. If brain is **affected** then romantic dream and liquid out **surely** while sleeping. Again keep it attention as any other people will not disturb you while you are doing love with your lover, if not it will affect to your brain.

You can keep love relation and sex relation with your lover, it is not a problem. But I want to solve your romantic dream and liquid out problem **completely**. It is possible to become curable from this disease **completely** within some days. If there is some **injury or infection or wound inside your brain** then you will see romantic dreams and liquid out while sleeping **surely.** So it is your work **to become curable** from this brain wound or infection or injury, then you will **never** see romantic dreams and no liquid out problem while sleeping. So it is your work **to take care** of your brain and **to keep safe** to your brain from any work pressure or any outside activities. It is **our aim** to keep safe to our brain. It is our **daily duty** and **daily work**. It is our daily work, it is our daily duty and it is our responsibility **to keep our brain safe** from different activities and outside activities. I can say that your romantic dream and liquid out problem while sleeping will be curable **completely** after reading this book. Then you will surely achieve the main aim, main goal of the human life before death.

Bad people are doing many preplanning to hurt to your mind and brain. Because they **can know** that if your brain will be affected then you will see romantic dreams and liquid out while sleeping. So they are hurting to your mind and brain by making different many **preplanning**. If you are looking too much dream while sleeping then there is another way to solve the problem of **too much dream** while sleeping. Get up early in the morning before sunrise, go to latrine then wash your hand, foot, face and mouth, then sit straight and comfortably on plain floor over a bed sheet in a room in your house for half an hour daily for some days. Then within some days this **too much dream** problem will be solved and you will not see too much dream.

It is our need to live in healthy and peaceful life. No one will interfere you in this way to live in healthy and happiness life. So try to become curable, try to become free from this romantic dreams and liquid out problem while sleeping. Then your whole life will be enjoyable **really**. So try to protect to your brain, try to keep safe to your brain. Then romantic dreams and liquid out problem will be solved **completely**.

Enemy tension is not the big tension, but try to **keep safe** to your brain. Try to keep safe to your brain from any type of work pressure. Try to keep safe to your brain form any romantic works. It is the **work**, it is the **duty**, it is **responsibility** of us **to keep safe** to our brain always form any type of outside activities. Then romantic dreams will not affect any bad and no liquid out while sleeping, if brain is safe.

All these thoughts of **romantic dreams** are also most useful to school, college students.

Always keep **attention** as anything will not affect to your brain. Always think about brain every day every moment as anything is **affected** to brain or not affected. Think about brain safety while going to bed while sleeping. Think **just before** sleeping that your brain is safe or not safe and think brain have any work pressure or free from work pressure. Then take special care while sleeping to sleep **full comfortably**. Always every moment think that brain is free from work pressure or not free. If you feel free in brain then it will be no romantic dream no liquid out while sleeping.

* * * * * * *

www.ingramcontent.com/pod-product-compliance
Lightning Source LLC
Chambersburg PA
CBHW040315240726
48664CB00006B/1497